THE TRIANGLE
MENTAL ILLNESS AND MENTAL WELLNESS

Understanding Schizophrenia, Bipolar Disorder, and Dementia; and Dealings with Patients Living with them.

Dr. Corie D. Johnson

Copyright © 2019

Copyright © 2019 Dr. Corie D. Johnson
All rights reserved.

All rights to this book are reserved. No permission is given for any part of this book to be reproduced, transmitted in any form or means; electronic or mechanical, stored in a retrieval system, photocopied, recorded, scanned, or otherwise. Any of these actions require the proper written permission of the publisher.

Disclaimer

All knowledge contained in this book is given for informational and educational purposes only. The author is not in any way accountable for any results or outcomes that emanate from using this material. Constructive attempts have been made to provide information that is both accurate and effective, but the author is not bound for the accuracy or use/misuse of this information.

Table of Contents

Introduction	1
Chapter One	**3**
Overview Of Mental Illness	3
Types of Mental Illness	4
Causes of Mental Illness	5
Symptoms Associated with Mental Illness	8
Prevention of Mental Illness	11
Chapter Two	**13**
Understanding Bipolar Disorder Or Manic Depression	13
What is Bipolar Disorder?	14
Types of Bipolar Disorder	15
Causes of Bipolar Disorder	17
Signs and Symptoms of Bipolar Disorder	18
Diagnosis of Bipolar Disorder	23
Treatment and Therapies for Bipolar Disorder	24
Chapter Three	**27**
Understanding Schizophrenia	27
What is Schizophrenia?	28
Causes of Schizophrenia	29
Symptoms of Schizophrenia	32
Symptoms in Teenagers	34
Complications of Schizophrenia	36
Diagnosis of Schizophrenia	36
Treatment and Therapies for Schizophrenia	38
Chapter Four	**41**
Understanding Dementia	41
What is Dementia?	42
Types of Dementia	43

CAUSES OF DEMENTIA	45
STAGES AND ASSOCIATED SYMPTOMS OF DEMENTIA	46
DIAGNOSIS OF DEMENTIA	48
EFFECTS OF DEMENTIA	49
THE CONTROL OF DEMENTIA	50

CHAPTER FIVE 52

TRANSFORMING MENTAL ILLNESS TO MENTAL WELLNESS	52
ACCEPTANCE	53
COMMUNICATION AND INTERACTION	55
MANAGEMENT AND CARE	56
RECOVERY	59

SUMMARY 60

Introduction

Mental health is crucial to the coordinative and cognitive well-being of human beings. When a human being experiences something other than this, they are said to be mentally ill. Mental illness comes in different forms and conditions. Do you know that mental illness is real, and happening to people around us? I know some of us here might be thinking that mental illness is something rare and uncommon in societies. If you are feeling this way, then I'm glad to let you know that mental illness is real, and it is common in people living around us. Do you know that an estimated 54 million Americans suffer from one form of mental disorder or another in a given year?

The sad thing is most people who have families living with one mental illness or the other are not well learned about the disease that the affected ones around them are facing, neither are prepared in any way to help their affected ones through the pathway of managing the mental illness and getting cures to the ones that can be healed. I would love to let you know that when you get the right knowledge to these diseases, you will understand how to deal and cope; which is why I have written this book. Understand your loved ones living around you; the symptoms they exhibit, and how to handle them when they show these features.

I would love you to understand that people affected by mental illness go through a hardship that they endure on a daily basis in their lives, getting proper understanding from people around them goes a long way, and you cannot care and love someone you do not correctly understand, or maybe I should put it in a better stance, that someone you are not prepared to understand. If you're interested in getting ready to understand and cope with their condition, the first step you need to take is read this book; the second step is to find a way to digest all you have read and apply to the real world around you.

The Journey is Eternal!

Chapter One
Overview Of Mental Illness

When anyone is ill, what do you say about them? You either say that they are sick, or they are not feeling well. When someone is mentally ill, the person is not operating in a state of mental well-being. Mental illness is a disease that ranges from mild to severe disturbances in thoughts coordination and behavioral patterns, which is not in line with the typical human mental structure, leading to inability to cope with life's ordinary demands and routines. Mental illness is a form of health condition that usually involves changes in behavior and way of thinking. This condition is also associated with distress and issues with functioning well at work, or in social or family activities.

We should know that many people living with one form of mental illness or the other usually don't want to disclose or talk about it to anyone. This is because people see mental illness as something stigmatizing, and shameful; but in the real sense, it is just a mental health condition that could receive medical attention, just like any other form of diseases that affects the human body. Mental illness doesn't discriminate; it can affect anyone irrespective of your age (it can occur at any age, most especially 3/4 of all mental disease start around age 24), gender, geographical location, income and social status, race/ethnicity, sexual orientation, religion/spirituality, or cultural identity.

It is essential for to know that mental illness is a common illness that affects people around us; some are evident while some are not. The thing is some people battle with one form of mental illness or another. It was recorded that in the United States at a given year that nearly one in five adults (which is equivalent to 19%) experience some form of mental illness; one in 24 (which is equal to 4.1%) has a severe mental illness; and one in 12 (which is equivalent to 8.5%) has a diagnosable substance use disorder. This shows that mental illness is something that is happening around us, and it is essential that we are aware of this fact. Many people around us have mental health issues frequently, but these issues result into mental illness when the signs and symptoms that they exhibit cause repetitive stress, which could affect the individual ability to function well in his/her normal state. This is to tell you that what they do well and effortlessly before it becomes somewhat tricky.

Mental illness usually occurs as a resultant effect from excessive stress generated from a particular situation or chain of events. Just like diabetes, cancer, and heart disease, mental illness is usually physical, emotional, and psychological. Mental illness may also be caused by a reaction to environmental stress, biochemical imbalances, and genetic factors; it could even be a combination of these. The state of mental illness is always challenging for those suffering it, as the disease could make them miserable and bring problems into their daily living; having to keep up with work, school, or even relationships with families, friends and loved ones become somewhat challenging. Although, some cases of mental illness can be treated and cured, some, however, can be managed through a combination of medications and talk therapy, which is also known as psychotherapy. When proper care is given, individuals living with the illness learn to cope with their condition and stay true to their journey to recovery from the mental illness.

Types of Mental Illness

There are over 200 types of mental illness. Common among them are Depression, Bipolar disorder, Dementia, Schizophrenia, Substance use disorder, Eating disorder, Autism Spectrum disorder, Post-Partum Depression, Posttraumatic stress disorder (PTSD), Obsessive-Compulsive Disorder (OCD), among many others. However, this book will look in depth into Bipolar disorder, Schizophrenia, and Dementia.

Causes of Mental Illness

Mental illness in different forms are caused by various factors in the genetic and environmental stance; this involves:

- **Inherited Traits:**

There is a form of gene inheritance between older generations with mental illness to the younger generation. What I am trying to say here is, when you have someone who is a relative battling with a form of mental illness, there is a possibility that another person in the bloodline, like the child, could inherit the same type of disease. This is because some specific genes may increase the risk of contracting the illness, and also life situations may trigger the effect.

- **Brain Chemistry:**

There is something we call the Neurotransmitters; they are naturally occurring brain chemicals that carry signals to the other parts of the human brain and the entire body. When there is an impairment in the neural networks involving these chemicals, the function of nerve receptors and nerve system changes, and this leads to depression in the human body.

- **Environmental Exposures before Birth:**

When a baby, while in the womb is exposed to some environmental stressors, inflammatory conditions, toxins, drugs, or alcohol; the baby has automatically been opened to the risk of having a mental illness when he/she is born. Proper care is always very essential while a mother is pregnant, so she doesn't expose the unborn child to a risk of having one form of mental illness or another.

There are other risk factors associated with mental illness which are outlined below:

- **Stressful life situations:** There are different things people face in life that brings mental illness to their body. For example, when a person who is doing well financially, suddenly run into an economic depression, it could lead the person to mental illness if proper precautions are not taken. Also, the death of a loved one so close, most notably the death of a husband or wife or children could lead people to mental illness. It is always advised that when people are faced with such situations in life, they should still have real companies around them without leaving them alone. Loneliness messes up their minds, and when a person's mind is messed up, mental illness is inevitable. Divorce is another situation that could lead one to a condition of mental illness.

- **Blood relative like parent or siblings with mental illness:** As I have discussed earlier, genetic inheritance occurs when a parent has the mental illness, children are always at a high risk of having the same mental illness; this because the mental illness is already in the bloodline.

- **Damages to the brain as a result of acute injury:** Brain damage caused as a result of injuries from either blows to the head, motor accident, could be responsible for mental illness. Some forms of Dementia like Parkinson's disease as a type of mental illness occur as a result of injuries that the brain has received during a cause of action. Street fighters and boxers are always at a risk of having mental illness due to the rigors of the game.

- **An ongoing chronic medical condition:** Some medical conditions at their chronic phase are always responsible for a state of mental illness. People with diabetes or cancer in their chronic phase often suffer some memory loss, which is a form of mental illness. This mental illness that they exhibit comes as a result of the chronic nature of the disease they process in their body.

- **Traumatic experiences:** People who have experienced some traumatic situations like assault, rape, or military combat are always at a risk of having Post Traumatic Stress Disorder (PTSD) which is a form of mental illness that is attributed to people who have been traumatized as a result of a bitter life experience that they have faced at a point in their lives.

- **Use of alcohol or drugs:** Habits they say die hard; when a person is given into a lifestyle of excessive drinking of alcohol, and indulgence in taking drugs like cocaine and heroin just to feel high. The resultant effect is that it leads them to a chronic mental disorder which if care is not taken could turn them to someone else entirely and lead them to the end of their lives. Always try as much as possible to run away from drugs, and make sure you indulge in taking too much alcohol. That would be good for your mental health.

- **Being abused or neglected as a child:** There are some experiences some people face in life that might seem like a something that shouldn't lead to mental illness, but the fact is they do and being neglected and abused as a child is one of them. Any child that has an abusive or neglected childhood usually have one form of mental disorder or the other. We must always listen to our children and not make them feel abandoned, we should also always shield them from any form of abuse, as this can traumatize their minds leading them to mental illness.

- **Having few friends or few healthy relationships:** This type of situation is always common among people who don't know how to socialize with people or people who are surrounded by negative minds and toxic relationships. When you are surrounded by negative and toxic people, your relationship with them is more toxic than not having friends at all. Relating with people like this will always have a negative effect on your mind; also when you have few friends, it might be more like being alone, and loneliness has a way of messing up someone's mind, mental illness at this point will occur. Surround yourselves with good people with a positive mindset, also make sure you make a new friend anytime you get to a new place.

- **A previous mental illness:** Having a previous mental illness can lead to another form of mental illness, or better still, the previous mental illness that was treated can reoccur if proper management practices are not put in place or observed. So, it is always good to avoid anything that could trigger the effects of a previous mental illness. Be watchful!

Symptoms Associated with Mental Illness

The signs and symptoms that come with mental illness vary, depending on the type of mental illness, the circumstances surrounding the mental illness, among other factors. The symptoms that come with mental illness have a way of affecting thoughts, emotions, and behaviors.

The symptoms of mental illness include the following:

- **Confused thinking or decline in the ability to concentrate:** When you notice your thought pattern is messed up or you realize that your ability to stay focused on something has reduced, I would advise you get yourself examined for mental illness as soon as possible.
- **Feeling sad or down:** This happens when you are always feeling unhappy, and nothing really gets you excited, and these anxious feelings will lead to depression. I will love you to seek medical advice if you are frequently feeling this way.

- **Extreme mood changes of highs and lows:** You are delighted this minute and feeling on top of the world; the next minute you are feeling extremely sad. These are mood irregularities that need medical attention.

- **Excessive fears or worries, feelings of guilt on the extreme:** Mental illness also comes with feeling fearful of small things and worrying excessively. Feeling incredibly guilty over matters that are dead and buried is also another symptom of mental illness. If you notice that you or your loved ones are feeling this way, I would advise you get medical help for proper examination.

- **Withdrawal from friends and activities:** Whenever you notice that your social life dropped and you don't get much excited at the company of family, friends and loved ones, and the excitement that comes with attending social functions have dropped drastically, then you should seek medical advice.

- **Detachment from reality (delusions), paranoia or hallucinations:** This symptom comes with having an image of things that are unreal, or unacceptable or inapplicable in the real world, having a feeling of people wanting to hurt you comes with this symptom too. When you exhibit this, I would advise you to seek the help of a medical expert.

- **Significant tiredness, low energy, or sleeping problems:** Getting tired quickly, having little power to work alongside problems with sleeping pattern can be attributed to mental illness, when this is noticed in you or your loved ones, get medical help.

- **Inability to cope with stress:** Here, we react gravely to the stress that we encounter in our daily lives, we find it difficult to deal with the challenges that come along with the task of each day. This is a symptom of mental illness, and it should be taken as a matter of seriousness.

- **Excessive anger, hostility or violence:** Mental illness comes with a sign getting angry unnecessarily, being hostile towards people around you, aggressiveness, and violence. You just have a feeling of wanting to react aggressively towards any uncomfortable happenings around you. When you notice that you are feeling this way, please consult a medical expert.

- **Trouble understanding and relating to situations and people:** The symptoms that come with mental illness involves finding it difficult to adequately assess conditions and understand people and the effect of action by people, this could be likened to confused thinking. Getting medical assistance is the best thing to do at this point.

- **Significant changes in eating habits:** People having irregular eating habits that involve loss of appetite, a sudden change in the choice of food, incompatible combination of diet and funny eating pattern should get conscious of the fact that they could be having a form of mental illness. Visiting the hospital for medical assessment is a viable option at this point.

- **Sex drive changes:** Mental illness also causes irregularities with libido. This involves loss of sex drive, and also there could be increased sex drive on the extreme. When this happens, you should be aware that it is beyond the usual human way of experiencing sex drive; this can be evidence of mental illness. Try and seek medical evaluation if you feel this way.

- **Alcohol or drug abuse:** Symptoms that comes with mental illness involves taking solace in taking alcohol excessively and also indulging in doing drugs, which in itself is a risk factor for mental illness. It is a symptom that comes with mental illness and in itself could make matters worse with the disease. When this is noticed, urgent action should be taken by visiting a medical expert.

- **Suicidal thinking:** Suicidal thoughts are always known with that mental illness, depression as a form of mental illness usually predisposes suicidal thoughts. When you notice that you or the people around you are getting suicidal in your way of thinking, talking, or actions; please, take urgent steps towards getting help through the right path. Meeting a medical expert or a psychologist is an excellent way to go.

Prevention of Mental Illness

Preventing mental illness does not go in a single specific way. There are different methods of preventing mental illness. If it happens that you are noticing the symptoms of mental illness in your body system, you need to take serious steps to control stress, increase your resilience, and try as much as possible to keep your self-esteem healthy and improved; it would also be good to keep the symptoms of the mental illness that you are experiencing under control. There are other steps you can follow, which includes the following:

- **Pay close attention to the warning signs:** You need to make sure you are working with your doctor or therapist to learn about the things that may trigger your symptoms. Develop a plan that would guide you on things to do if symptoms return. Try and contact your doctor or therapist if you notice any changes in symptoms or how you feel. Consider involving family members or friends to watch out for warning signs.
- **Get routine medical care:** Always go for medical checkups from time to time. Don't skip your visit to your health care provider, most especially if you are not feeling well. Visiting from time to time will make you understand how your body works because you will get to ask questions on any development of a new health prob-

lem you noticed in your body; clarification on it could show whether it is a side effect from a medication.

- **Get help in the times you need help:** Don't wait till things get out of hand before you request for help. Mental illness could grow worse and become harder to treat if timely actions are not taken towards getting treated. Also, long-term maintenance of the illness may help to relapse the effect of the symptoms.

- **Take proper care of yourself:** This involves you imbibing good habits that will make you always healthy. This consists of getting sufficient sleep, eating healthy, regular physical activity, and avoiding unnecessary stress. Maintain a routine, communicate with your health care provider if you any issues, and seek instructions on diet and physical activities.

Chapter Two
Understanding Bipolar Disorder or Manic Depression

When you are talking about a condition that shows extreme shifts in mood and fluctuations in energy and activity levels that can make day-to-day living challenging, then you can talk about Bipolar Disorder. During the phases of the illness, there are different sessions of depression, the conditions may come with crying, and their outlook on life changes from being favorable to negativity; they also have poor eye contact with people at the periods of this disease. Bipolar disorder can be so deadly to the extent that it could lead those affected to committing suicide. Individuals with this disease usually make poor thought decisions with little regards to the consequences of their actions.

The risk of committing suicide among those living with bipolar disorder is high at greater than 6% over 20 years, while self-harm occurs in 30-40% of those living with the disease. Other mental illnesses are associated with bipolar disorder, which includes anxiety disorders and attention-deficit hyperactivity disorder (ADHD). Substance use disorder involves the misuse of alcohol or drugs, people with substance abuse disorder usually have relationship problems, they don't perform well in school or at work, family, friends, and people experiencing symptoms may not recognize these problems as signs of a significant mental illness, which is also familiar with bipolar disorder.

Bipolar disorder affects approximately 1% of the world population. In the United States, about 3% are assessed to be concerned with bipolar disorder at some point in their life; rates appear to be similar in females and males. The most common age when the symptoms of the bipolar disorder begin is at 25. The economic cost of the disease has been estimated at $45 billion for the United States in 1991. A large amount of this was related to a higher number of missed workdays, determined at 50 per year. People with bipolar disorder often face issues with social stigma, and this, at some point, doesn't usually make them want to seek medical attention.

What is Bipolar Disorder?

Bipolar disorder, formerly known as manic depression, is a mental illness that causes periods of depression and periods of abnormally elevated moods. What we are saying here is people living with the bipolar disease have abnormalities in their mood pattern, they are highly elated this minute, and the next they are gravely sad. They experience alternating episodes of extreme euphoria, or mania, and major depression. There is severity in the fluctuations that they experience, but their moods may be normal between the peaks and troughs. The mood swings involved in bipolar disorder are far more severe, devastating, and weakening than other mental illnesses experienced by most people.

The severity of mood episodes can vary from very mild to extreme, and they can occur steadily or swiftly within a timeframe of days to weeks. When isolated mood episodes happen four or more times per year, the process is known as rapid cycling. Rapid cycling should not be confused with very recurrent moment-to-moment changes in mood, which can occasionally occur in people living with bipolar disorder or other conditions such as borderline personality disorder. When a person living with bipolar become depressed, they may feel sad or hopeless and lose interest or pleasure in most activities. They experience mood shifts to mania or hypomania (less extreme than mania), which makes them feel euphoric, full of energy or bizarrely irritable. These mood swings can affect sleep, energy, activity, judgment, behavior and the ability to think clearly.

Bipolar disorder occurs with episodes of mood swings, which may happen rarely or multiple times a year. While most people will experience some emotional symptoms between episodes, some may not experience any. Although bipolar disorder is a lifelong mental health condition, you can manage your mood swings and other symptoms by following a treatment plan. In most cases, bipolar disorder can be treated with medicinal prescriptions and psychological counselling (psychotherapy).

Types of Bipolar Disorder

Bipolar disorder comes in four primary forms, of which all of them shows evident changes in mood, energy, and activity levels. These changes in attitudes vary from periods of extremely 'up', exhilarated and energized feelings also known as Manic Episodes; to periods of very sad, 'down', or hopeless feelings also known as Depressive Episodes. The less severe manic periods are also known as Hypomanic Episodes. The four types of bipolar disorder include the following:

> ➤ **Bipolar I Disorder:**
>
> This form of the disease is known for manic episodes that last at least seven days, or by manic symptoms that are severe to the extent that the person needs immediate hospital care. People living with this type of disorder must have had at least one manic episode that may go before or followed by hypomanic or major depressive episodes. In some cases, mania may activate a break from reality (psychosis). The depressive episodes in this form of the disorder usually take place and lasting not less than two weeks. Episodes of depression with mixed characters (having depression and manic symptoms at the same time) are also likely.

- **Bipolar II Disorder:**

    Bipolar II Disorder is defined by a form of depressive episodes and hypomanic episodes, but not the full-blown manic episodes as described in bipolar I disorder. For a diagnosis of bipolar II, the patient must have experienced one or more episodes of depression, and at least one hypomanic episode. The hypomanic state in bipolar II disorder is less severe than the manic state. Hypomanic episodes involve less sleep, competitiveness, outgoing and energy-filled nature. People exhibiting these episodes function in their full quality, which differs from the case with manic episodes. Bipolar II can also involve mixed episodes, and there may be symptoms of mood-congruent or mood-incongruent psychotic features. A mood-congruent psychosis would include features that match the mood. For instance, if a person is suffering from depression, mood-congruent psychosis could have a tone of sadness.

- **Cyclothymic Disorder:**

    Cyclothymic disorder, also known as Cyclothymia is known for its nature of having numerous periods of hypomanic symptoms as well multiple periods of depressive symptoms lasting for at least two years (1 year in children and adolescents). However, the signs do not meet the diagnostic requirements for a hypomanic episode and a depressive episode.

- **Other types:**

    Other types of bipolar disorder include bipolar and other related mental illness that is induced by certain drugs or alcohol, or as a result of a medical condition, such as Cushing's disease, multiple sclerosis or stroke.

Causes of Bipolar Disorder

The roots of bipolar disorder do not appear to be farfetched, as it does not seem to have a single purpose, there is a likeliness of it to result from a range of contributory factors, and this includes:

Genetic Factors

It has been suggested from myriads of research that people with some peculiar genes are more likely to develop bipolar disorder than others. But genes are not the only risk factor for bipolar disorder. Studies conducted on identical twins showed that even if one twin develops bipolar disorder at some point in life, the other twin does not have to develop the disorder even though identical twins share all of the same genes. There is an association of bipolar disorder with the reduced manifestation of specific DNA repair enzymes and increased levels of oxidative DNA damages. I hope I have not confused you with scientific languages yet. Let me add this here that advanced has been connected to a somewhat increased chance of bipolar disorder in offspring, consistent with a hypothesis of increased new genetic mutation.

Brain Structure and Functioning

Some studies show the way the brains of people with bipolar disorder operates may differ from the way the brains of healthy people or people with other mental disorder works. When we learn more about these differences, along with new information from genetic studies, we get to understand the bipolar disorder better and predict the types of treatment that will be most effective. Looking at it from the neurological angle, bipolar disorder may occur as a result of neurological condition or injury, which could be in the form of stroke, porphyria, traumatic brain injury, multiple sclerosis, among others.

Environmental Factors

Environmental factors, which could also be seen in a psychosocial form, plays a significant role in the development of a bipolar disorder, and even psychosocial variables may relate with genetic natures. The experience that people encounter in their relationships with people and the environment contribute to the recurrence of bipolar mood episodes. Recent surveys have shown that 30-50% of adults diagnosed with bipolar disorder report traumatic and abusive experiences in their childhood, and this could be related to the higher rates of suicide attempts and other co-occurring disorder such as post-traumatic stress disorder (PTSD). The number of successful events in childhood that is recorded is higher in those with an adult diagnosis of bipolar spectrum disorder when compared to those without; which also be traced from an unfriendly environment preferably from the child's behavior.

Signs and Symptoms of Bipolar Disorder

The signs and symptoms associated with bipolar disorder vary between people, and according to the mood. Some people have distinctive mood swings, with symptoms of mania and then of depression, which could last several months or months of stability between them. Some people spend months or years experiencing a 'high' or 'low' mood. The symptoms of bipolar come with the different episodes of hypomania and mania, which are further discussed below.

Mania Signs in Bipolar Disorder

The mania signs of bipolar disorder include the following:

- **Disconnected and swift (racing) thoughts:** Have you ever tried to see a movie and you decide to do a fast forward of some scenes a couple of times? The fast movement of the video can be likened to the thinking pattern of people with bipolar disorder experiencing mania. Their thoughts follow a distorted model, of which putting the thoughts together wouldn't make too much sense.

- **Grandiose beliefs:** The sign of mania comes with planning or trying to figure out something unrealistic and unattainable. People experiencing mania are unnecessarily confident that they can on their do what will take up to seven people to do effectively. An instance is someone believing he can lift a heavy machine that would involve four able-bodied men for a successful lifting. People like that don't want to consider they are old even when they are old in the real sense.

- **Inappropriate elation or euphoria:** This involves an experience of great excitement at things that are not so enchanting in the real sense. They are usually unable to control how they feel or even control their tongue, and they say what they are not supposed to say out of joy.

- **Inappropriate irritability:** The mania symptoms conjure to the fact that the sense of responsibility to stimuli becomes distorted. The response at this point is usually incoherent with the situation or sequence of events.

- **Inappropriate social behavior:** The social actions that people with mania exhibits are generally inappropriate; this may be due to the hyper nature of their condition. Social vices like fighting, excessive alcohol, and drug abuse are inevitable from people at this episode of bipolar disorder. Talking too much is also another significant sign that comes with this.

- **Increased sexual desire:** The libido experienced at this episode is somewhat crazy. They tend not to get satisfied anymore with sex from a single partner, and they thereby go-ahead to explore sex from multiple sexual partners.

- **Increased talking speed or volume:** Due to the way their brain works, remember we talked about the mania symptoms coming with racing thoughts; the thing is the racing thoughts usually transcend to the increased talking speed of the patients exhibiting mania.
- **Markedly increased energy:** The high mood that comes with the mania symptoms also shows a remarkable energized nature making you feel you can do anything. You feel like Superhero.
- **Poor judgment:** Since the thought pattern of those exhibiting mania episodes of the bipolar disorder become distorted, the sense of judgment of such people becomes incredibly poor.
- **A decreased need for sleep due to high energy:** The hyper or "Superhero" energy that is exhibited takes away sleep. The funny thing here is it doesn't feel as if sleep is needed.

Hypomania Signs in Bipolar II Disorder

The signs that are exhibited in hypomania are somewhat similar to those of mania, and they are outlined below:

- **Decreased need for sleep:** As discussed earlier, insomnia is usually attached to the signs of hypomania due to high mood.
- **Extreme focus on projects at work or home:** The high energy brings out the workaholic in the sense that you channel those energies to projects at work such that you don't even know when to draw the line between home and work. You work everywhere.
- **Exuberant and happy mood:** At this episode, you exhibit some unusual and over-joyous mood, which could be inappropriate.

- **Increased confidence:** This comes with you crazily believing yourself that you can do anything. Like I discussed earlier, it brings the Superhero out of you.
- **Increased creativity and productivity:** When the high energy is channeled into working, definitely there will be increased creativity and productivity. However, the excessiveness will show that it is a form of the disorder that is being exhibited.
- **Increased energy and libido:** The sex drive is increased, and your hunger for sex becomes insatiable, leading to you to having multiple sexual partners.
- **Reckless behaviors:** The high energy in this episode can be translated into indulging in careless and reckless acts. Such as alcoholism and drug abuse, which could lead to other vices.
- **Risky pleasure-seeking behaviors:** The hyper nature of this symptoms would always make those affected with hypomania want to try out some pleasurable activities that could be risky for their health, and also cause physical harm to the body.

Depressive Symptoms of Bipolar Disorder

The depressive episode of bipolar disorder is most terrible and more deadly than the earlier discussed phases. Outlined below are the symptoms that could be exhibited from the depressive phase:

- **Feeling of gloom, blackness, despair, and hopelessness:** This is a crazy feeling that makes you feel like nothing good can come out of you. Just an exact opposite of the mania episodes of bipolar disorder. It comes with a total loss of hope over oneself or a situation.

- **Extreme sadness:** Generally, depression comes with extreme sadness. It is always a down mood for those exhibiting the depressive symptom of bipolar disorder.

- **Insomnia and sleeping problems:** They lose their sleep easily at this phase because they are too sad to the thoughts, their hearts become burdensome, and sleep becomes almost impossible.

- **Anxiety about trivial things:** These symptoms come with getting unnecessarily worked up over small and unimportant issues. It involves carrying the burden in the heart and refusing to let go.

- **Pain or physical problems that do not respond to treatment:** Due to the depressive nature of this episode, depression in itself usually brings forward different forms of diseases, and when these diseases surface, they are generally challenging to dismiss. This is because depression in itself is the actual fueling force for diseases to thrive.

- **Guilt, and a feeling that everything that goes wrong or appears to be wrong is their fault:** As funny as it is, what should have been dead and forgotten begins to resurface, because the memory of the negative events that are experienced in the past are being replaced by the depressive nature of the bipolar disorder.

- **Changes in eating patterns, whether eating more or eating less:** Distorted eating habits are usually known for people living with depressive bipolar disorder. Either not having an appetite for food, or have unnecessary cravings, and overeating.

- **Weight loss or weight gain:** Taking a cue from the previous point, not eating well, definitely will show a loss in weight, and also carelessly and excessively eating tends to gain much weight. These symptoms come with the depressive episode.

- **Extreme tiredness, fatigue, and listlessness:** Getting tired easily and reduced zeal to work comes from the depressive symptoms of bipolar disorder. A person that is depressed is usually laid back from doing work. This is because the unhappy nature drains a lot of energy from them. Hope you dig.
- **An inability to enjoy activities or interests that usually give pleasure:** A depressed person will never want to engage in any lively activities, typically do not see any actual reason for them to take a time out and have fun.
- **Low attention span and difficulty remembering:** Depressed people generally are easily carried away with their mind, not within their immediate environment. Also, putting things to account becomes a difficult task.
- **Irritation, possibly triggered by noises, smells, tight clothing, and other things that would usually be tolerated or ignored:** They typically get irritated easily by things that are seen as being normal. They get gravely irritated by noise, smells (even fragrances), and tight clothing, and even food aroma.
- **An inability to face going to work or school, possibly leading to underperformance:** The depressive nature usually leads to lack of confidence in one's self and in that sense, motivation goes down, and lack of motivation will affect productivity at work or in school.

Diagnosis of Bipolar Disorder

As with most mood disorders, there are no laboratory tests or brain imaging method to diagnose bipolar disorder. Just like dementia, after performing a physical exam, your doctor will evaluate your signs and symptoms. Your doctor will also ask you about your personal medical history and family history.

Lab tests may be done to rule out other medical illnesses that can affect mood.

Also, your doctor may want to talk with family members to see if they can identify times when you were elated and over-energized. Because elation may feel good or even healthy when compared to depression, it's often hard for a person with bipolar disorder to know if the mood was too high. Mania usually affects thinking, judgment, and social behavior in ways that cause serious problems and embarrassment. For example, unwise business or financial decisions may be made when an individual is in a manic phase. So early diagnosis and effective treatment are vital with bipolar disorder.

Treatment and Therapies for Bipolar Disorder

The treatment and therapies for bipolar disorder aim to minimize the frequency of manic and depressive episodes and to decrease the severity of symptoms to facilitate a relatively productive and healthy life. If left untreated, a session of depression or mania can persist for up to 1 year. But with treatment, you should be sure that improvements are possible within 3 to 4 months.

The treatment for bipolar disorder involves a combination of therapies, which may include medications and physical and psychological interventions. The person may continue to experience mood changes, but working closely with a doctor can reduce the severity and make the symptoms more manageable.

Drug treatment

Lithium carbonate is the most generally prescribed long-term drug to treat long-term episodes of depression and mania or hypomania. Patients usually take lithium for at least six months. It is essential for the patient to follow the doctor's instructions about when and how to take their medication to ensure the drugs to work.

Other treatments include:

- **Anticonvulsants:** These are sometimes prescribed to treat mania episodes.
- **Antipsychotics:** Aripiprazole, olanzapine, risperidone are some of the options if the behavior is very disturbed and symptoms are severe.

Medication may need to be adjusted as moods shift, and some drugs have side effects. Some antidepressants given to patients before they have a diagnosis of bipolar disorder may trigger a first manic episode. A physician who is treating a patient with depression should monitor for this.

Psychotherapy, CBT, and Hospitalization

Psychotherapy aims to alleviate and help the patient manage the symptoms that come with bipolar disorder. If the patient can identify and recognize the key triggers, they may be able to minimize the secondary effects of the condition.

The person can learn to recognize the first symptoms that indicate the onset of an episode and work on the factors that can help maintain the "normal" periods for as long as possible. This can help maintain positive relationships at home and work. So, the wife/husband, kids, and friends can enjoy having you around them.

Cognitive behavioral therapy (CBT), as an individual or family-focused treatment, can also help avert relapses. Interpersonal and social rhythm therapy, combined with CBT, can also help with depressive symptoms.

Hospitalization is not as frequent now as it was in the past. However, brief hospitalization may be advisable if there is a risk of the patient harming themselves or others. Electroconvulsive therapy (ECT) may help if other treatments are not sufficient.

Keeping up a routine with a healthy diet, enough sleep, and regular exercise can help the person maintain stability. Any supplements should first be discussed with a doctor, as some alternative remedies can interact with the drugs used for bipolar disorder or exacerbate symptoms.

Chapter Three
Understanding Schizophrenia

Taking time to understand schizophrenia will make us know the depth of its severity. Schizophrenia is a chronic mental illness that affects not just the old but also the younger adults, in that it appears in late adolescence or early adulthood. People with schizophrenia usually experience hallucination, delusions, and other cognitive difficulties. This mental illness can be a life long struggle in the sense that people with schizophrenia require lifelong treatment. Early treatment may help to put the symptoms under control before serious complications develop and may help improve the long-term outlook.

Schizophrenia is a mental illness characterized by abnormal behavior, strange speech, and a decreased ability to understand reality. Other symptoms include false beliefs, unclear or confused thinking, hearing voices that do not exist, reduced social engagement and emotional expression, and lack of motivation to get things done. People living with schizophrenia often have additional problems, which include anxiety, substance-use disorder, and depression, among others. Schizophrenia does not imply a "split personality" or dissociative identity disorder, conditions with which it is often confused in public perception.

Around 1% of the world's population is affected by schizophrenia during their lifetimes. In 2013, there were an estimated 23.6 million cases globally. Males are more often affected and on average experience more severe symptoms. About 20% of people eventually do well, and a few recover completely. About 50% have permanent damage. Social problems, such as long-term unemployment, poverty, and homelessness, are common. The average life expectancy of people with the disorder is 10–25 years less than that of the general population. This is the result of increased physical health problems and a higher suicide rate (about 5%). In 2015, an estimated 17,000 people worldwide died from behavior that is concerning, or caused by, schizophrenia. Experts have seen schizophrenia as many illnesses masquerading as one.

What is Schizophrenia?

Schizophrenia is a severe mental disorder that affects the way a person thinks, feels, and behaves. It is a mental illness that distorts the thought pattern and behavioral pattern of the people living with the disease. People with schizophrenia may seem like they have lost touch with reality. Although schizophrenia is not as common as other mental disorders, the symptoms can be debilitating.

This mental illness called schizophrenia is a chronic brain disorder that affects less than 1% of the population of the United States. When schizophrenia becomes active in people, the symptoms that they exhibit include delusions, hallucinations, trouble with thinking and concentration, and lack of motivation. However, with treatment, there could be a significant improvement in the most symptoms of schizophrenia.

It has been shown from research that schizophrenia affects men and women in almost equal proportions, but the thing is, it may have an earlier onset in males. The rates of this ailment are quite similar around the world. People with schizophrenia are more likely to die younger than the general population, in part because of high rates of co-occurring medical conditions, such as heart disease and diabetes, of which these are life-threatening in themselves.

The complexity that comes with schizophrenia may help explain the reasons for the different misconceptions about the disease. Schizophrenia does not imply a split personality or multiple personality. We should know this for a truth that most people living with schizophrenia are not dangerous or violent; they also are not homeless neither do they live in hospitals. Most people that have schizophrenia live with family, in group homes or on their own. In as much as we see mental illness as chronic, we should not allow the misconceptions that comes with it rule our being and determine our attitude towards people living with such mental health challenge.

While it seems like there is no cure for schizophrenia, optimized research is on and leading to new, safer treatments. Experts also are unravelling the causes of the disease by studying genetics, conducting behavioral analysis, and using advanced imaging to look at the brain's structure and function. These approaches hold the promise of new, more effective therapies.

Causes of Schizophrenia

The roots of schizophrenia do not take a specific clarification, but it has been reasoned out by the researchers the possible causes of the mental illness which are discussed below:

> **Genetic Inheritance**

  The family connection to the disease is an essential cause in this stance. If there it happens that there is no history of schizophrenia in a family, then the chances of developing the disease are less than 1%. However, that risk of having schizophrenia rises to 10% if a parent was diagnosed. It is no more news for scientists, as it has been known for a while now that schizophrenia sometimes runs in families. However, many people have schizophrenia and do not have a family member with the disorder, and conversely, there are many people with one or more family members with the disease who do not develop it themselves. Scientists believe that many different genes may increase the risk of schizophrenia, but no single gene causes the disorder by itself. It is not yet possible to use genetic information to predict who will develop schizophrenia.

It was estimated that the heritability of schizophrenia is around 80%, and this implies that 80% of the individual differences in risk to schizophrenia is associated with genetics. These estimates vary because of the difficulty in separating genetic and environmental influences. The maximum single risk factor for developing schizophrenia has a first-degree relative with the disease (the risk is 6.5%); more than 40% of monozygotic twins of those with schizophrenia are also affected. If one parent is affected, the risk has schizophrenia about 13%, and if both are affected, the risk is nearly 50%. Results of candidate gene studies of schizophrenia have generally failed to find harmonious relations, and the genetic loci identified by genome-wide association studies as associated with schizophrenia explain only a tiny fraction of the disparity in the disease.

➢ Environment

Environmental factors that are related to the development of schizophrenia include the living environment, drug use, and prenatal stressors.

Maternal stress has been associated with an increased risk of schizophrenia. This could be in the form of maternal nutritional deficiencies, such as those observed during a famine, as well as maternal obesity, have also been recognized as possible risk factors for schizophrenia.

Parenting style seems to have no significant effect on schizophrenia, although, people with supportive parents do better than those with critical or hostile parents. Childhood trauma, death of a parent, and being bullied or abused increase the risk of psychosis. Living in an urban environment during childhood or as an adult has consistently been found to increase the risk of schizophrenia as a factor, even after taking into account drug use, ethnic group, and size of a social group. Other factors that play an important role include social isolation and immigration related to social adversity, racial discrimination, family dysfunction, unemployment, and poor housing conditions.

➢ Substance Use

It has been asserted that about half of those with schizophrenia use drugs or alcohol excessively. Amphetamine, cocaine, and to lesser extent, alcohol, can result in a transient stimulant psychosis or alcohol-related psychosis that presents very similarly to schizophrenia. Although it is not generally believed to be a cause of the illness, people with schizophrenia use nicotine at much higher rates than the general population.

Alcohol abuse can occasionally cause the development of a chronic, substance-induced psychotic disorder via a kindling mechanism. Alcohol use is not associated with an earlier onset of psychosis. Cannabis may be a contributory factor in schizophrenia, potentially causing the disease in those who are already at risk. The increased risk may require the presence of specific genes within an individual. Among those who are at risk of psychosis, it is associated with twice the rate. Other drugs may be used only as coping mechanisms by people who have schizophrenia, to deal with depression, anxiety, boredom, and loneliness.

➢ Chemical Imbalance in the Brain

Experts believe that disproportion of dopamine, a neurotransmitter, plays a vital role in the onset of schizophrenia. Other neurotransmitters, such as serotonin, may also be involved.

Symptoms of Schizophrenia

Quite a sizable proportion of people with schizophrenia have to rely on others because they are unable to hold a job or care for themselves or others. Many may also resist treatment, arguing that there is nothing wrong with them. Some patients may show apparent symptoms, but on other occasions, they may seem fine until they begin to explain what they are honestly thinking. The effects of schizophrenia reach far beyond the patient - families, friends, and society are affected too. Symptoms and signs of schizophrenia will vary, depending on the individual.

The symptoms are classified into the following proportions:

> **Positive Symptoms:**

The positive symptoms of schizophrenia come with psychotic behaviors that are not generally noticed in healthy people. The people having these positive symptoms may lose touch with some parts of real-time experiences. The positive signs likened to schizophrenia includes the following:

- **Delusions:** The feeling of delusion involves the patient displaying false beliefs, which can take many forms, such as delusions of persecution, or delusions of grandeur. They may feel others are attempting to control them remotely. They may also think that they have extraordinary powers and abilities.

- **Hallucinations:** This involves hearing voices that are not real, much more common than seeing, feeling, tasting, or smelling things which are not there, however, people with schizophrenia may experience a wide range of hallucinations.

- **Thought Disorders:** People having thought disorder usually jump from one subject of conversation to another for no logical reason. This makes it hard to follow through with the discussion of the person living with this mental illness. People around them could even consider them as being erratic.

- **Movement Disorders:** Movement disorder here refers to people with schizophrenia walking in a distorted manner, and also exhibiting a lousy walking posture, this usually makes the people around patients living with schizophrenia notice more that something is wrong when it is not yet evident.

➢ **Negative Symptoms:**

The negative symptoms of schizophrenia are associated with disruptions to normal emotions and behaviors. The symptoms that come with it includes the following:

- **Difficulty beginning and sustaining activities:** The experiences involve finding it challenging to embark on tasks. People living with this illness are usually not organized, difficulties in maintaining activities.

- **Reduced speaking:** This comes with slowness in speaking, and even at times, you don't want to engage in long conversations. It could also involve unnecessary quietness.

- **Reduced feelings of pleasure in everyday life**: At this point, you don't feel so excited about things that bring fun to a normal human being. Going out for fun trips, parties, and other social functions does not excite you anymore. You'd instead prefer to stay back home and be on your own.

- **Flat affect:** This happens when there is a reduced expression of emotions through voice tone and facial expression. Their attitudes show that they are less emotional about things happening in their surroundings.

➢ **Cognitive Symptoms:**

The cognitive symptoms of schizophrenia for some patients are somewhat subtle, but for others, are more severe, patients may notice changes in their memory or other aspects of thinking and mental coordination. The cognitive symptoms that come with schizophrenia include the following:

- **Trouble focusing or paying attention:** The cognitive trait here shows that people living with schizophrenia often find it difficult to concentrate on a thing for a long time. The issue here is as a result of the instability of the mind structure.

- **Challenges with working memory:** People with schizophrenia exhibit this symptom often find it challenging to apply the things that they have learned into productive action. This is because they tend to forget what they have learned so quickly.

- **Poor executive functioning:** This symptom involves the inability to properly understand the information given for a course of action, which will, in turn, affect a proper sense of decision making. Cognitive impairment makes it difficult to process the information provided for decision making. Also, resulting in low productivity because the right decision might not be made.

Symptoms in Teenagers

The symptoms of schizophrenia in teenagers are similar to those in adults, but the illness may be more challenging to recognize. This may be in part because some of the early symptoms of schizophrenia in teenagers are collective for healthy development during teen years, such as:

- **Withdrawal from friends and family:** Here, they want to leave the company of people no matter how close to them and take solace in being on their own. This, however, should not be allowed as it can trigger the symptoms to become more severe and also bring forth additional signs when proper is not taken.

- **A drop in performance at school:** One of the things that you notice about them is that the academic performance of the young folks living with schizophrenia begins to drop. This may be as a result of the lack of motivation among other cognitive impairments that comes with the mental illness.

- **Trouble sleeping:** Insomnia is another sign that comes with schizophrenia. The sleeping pattern becomes distorted as they regularly experience loss of sleep. This is unhealthy, and it could give way to other additional health challenges.

- **Irritability or depressed mood:** People with schizophrenia get unnecessarily irritated by foods, noises, and other things that are appreciated in healthy people. They also get depressed and depression is indeed dangerous as it could lead to suicide.

- **Lack of motivation:** This involves people having schizophrenia losing the required drive to get something done. The push is no more there, and they become laid back when it comes to getting tasks done. The resultant effect of this is poor delivery.

Compared with schizophrenia symptoms in adults, teens may be:

- **Less likely to have delusions:** Delusion involves in having a belief in something somewhat superstitious, and also displaying a false belief. And these are usually not common with the younger folks. It is more prevalent among adults and seniors.

- **More likely to have visual hallucinations:** Visual hallucinations involve having an image of something unreal. Healthy people don't get to see and feel what people living with schizophrenia see and feel. Visual hallucinations are more common among younger folks than among the older adults and seniors.

Complications of Schizophrenia

When schizophrenia is left untreated, it can result in severe problems, and these problems can affect every area of life. Complications that schizophrenia may cause or be associated with include:

- Suicide, suicide attempts and thoughts of suicide.
- Self-injury.
- Anxiety disorders and obsessive-compulsive disorder (OCD).
- Depression.
- Abuse of alcohol or other drugs, including tobacco.
- Inability to work or attend school.
- Legal and financial problems and homelessness.
- Social isolation.
- Health and medical problems.
- Being victimized.
- Aggressive behavior, although it's uncommon.

Diagnosis of Schizophrenia

The diagnosis of schizophrenia is reached by noticing the actions of the patient. If the doctor suspects the possibility of schizophrenia, they will proceed to get to know about the patient's medical and psychiatric history. Specific tests will be directed by the doctors to rule out other illnesses and conditions that may be a trigger for schizophrenia-like symptoms. These tests include:

- **Blood tests:** This is usually done in cases where drug use may be a factor. The blood test may be ordered to know the presence and extent of the drug use in the body system. Blood tests are also done to exclude physical causes of illness.
- **Imaging studies:** This is done to rule out tumors and problems in the structure of the brain.
- **Psychological evaluation:** This form of assessment is done by a specialist, who will assess the patient's mental state by asking about thoughts, moods, hallucinations, suicidal traits, violent tendencies, or potential for violence, as well as observing their demeanor and appearance.

Schizophrenia Diagnosis Criteria

For a person to have schizophrenia, he/she must have met the requirements outlined in the DSM (Diagnostic and Statistical Manual of Mental Disorders). In case you are wondering what that is all about; DSM is an American Psychiatric Association manual used by healthcare professionals to diagnose mental illnesses and conditions. There is a need for doctors to exclude other possible mental health disorders, such as bipolar disorder or schizoaffective disorder.

It is also essential to establish that a prescribed medication or substance abuse have not caused the signs and symptoms.

The patient must have at least two of the following typical symptoms:

- Hallucinations.
- Delusions.
- Disorganized speech.

- Disorganized or catatonic behavior.
- Negative symptoms that are present for much of the time during the last four weeks.
- Experience significant impairment in the ability to attend school, carry out their work duties, or carry out everyday tasks.
- Have symptoms that persist for six months or more.

Treatment and Therapies for Schizophrenia

When people with schizophrenia are appropriately treated, they can lead productive lives; so, writing off a person living with mental illness is not an option here. Treatment can help relieve many of the symptoms of schizophrenia. However, most of the patients living with the disorder may have to cope with the symptoms for life. Psychiatrists say the most effective treatment for schizophrenia patients is usually a combination of:

- Medication
- Psychological counselling
- Self-help resources

Anti-psychosis drugs have transformed schizophrenia treatment. Thanks to them, most patients can live in the community, rather than stay in a hospital.

The most common schizophrenia medications are:

- **Risperidone (Risperdal):** This medication less sedating than other atypical antipsychotics. Weight gain and diabetes are possible side effects, but are less likely to happen, compared with Clozapine or Olanzapine.

- **Olanzapine (Zyprexa):** This may also improve negative symptoms. However, the risks of serious weight gain and the development of diabetes are significant.
- **Quetiapine (Seroquel):** The risk of weight gain and diabetes is also posed with this medication. However, the risk is lower than Clozapine or Olanzapine.
- **Ziprasidone (Geodon):** The risk of weight gain and diabetes with this medication is lower than other atypical antipsychotics. However, it might contribute to cardiac arrhythmia.
- **Clozapine (Clozaril):** This medication is useful for patients who have been resistant to treatment. It is known to lower suicidal behaviors in patients with schizophrenia. The risk of weight gain and diabetes is significant.
- **Haloperidol:** This medication is an antipsychotic used in the treatment of schizophrenia. It has proven to have a long-lasting effect (weeks).

The primary treatment for schizophrenia is medication. Conversely, compliance (following the medication regimen) is a significant problem, and that's quite disappointing because it doesn't bring forth the efforts the health care providers are putting in place to get them in a good state of well-being. People with schizophrenia often come off their medication for long periods during their lives, at enormous personal costs to themselves and often to those around them. It is essential here to watch your loved ones living with schizophrenia closely and make sure they are using their medication from time to time. The patient must continue taking medication even when symptoms are not present. Otherwise, there is a profound possibility that the illness will come back.

The first time a person experiences schizophrenia symptom, it can be extremely unpleasant. They may take a long time to recover, and that recovery can be a lonely experience. It is crucial that a person living with schizophrenia receives the full support of their family, friends, and community services when onset appears for the first time. Care, support and understanding at that point in their lives goes a long way towards the healing and coping process of the mental illness.

Chapter Four
Understanding Dementia

When you hear of the disease called dementia, there should be a couple of things you must keep in view; the source of the disease, the extent of the disease and those affected the most by the disease. Moving on from there, we can describe dementia as a large class of mental illness that results to a long-term and usually a gradual decrease in the ability to put your thoughts together, which in turns affects the daily functioning of the affected person. Dementia involves a decline in the mental functioning of a person from the usual way of the proper functioning of the brain. This is what happens when you have a person who is known to be sound in reasoning suddenly or gradually begins to have an uncoordinated reasoning pattern, which will also affect some other parts of the body that will be further discussed under the section of the symptoms involved with dementia.

Globally, dementia affected about 46 million people in 2015. About 10% of people have a disorder at some point in their lives. Dementia becomes more common with age as it is a disease that is common amongst seniors. About 3% of people between the ages of 65–74 have dementia, 19% between 75 and 84, and nearly half of those over 85 years of age. In 2013, dementia resulted in about 1.7 million deaths up from 8 million in 1990. The longer people live, the more the mental illness called dementia becomes common in the population. For people of a specific age, however, it may be becoming less frequent, at least in the developed world, due to a decrease in risk factors. It is one of the most common causes of disability amongst older people. It is believed to result in economic costs of US 604 billion a year. People with dementia are often physically or chemically restrained to a higher degree than necessary, raising issues of human rights. Social stigma against those affected is prevalent. We should also know this for the fact that some of the symptoms that come with dementia occur similarly in other mental illness, including schizophrenia and bipolar disorder.

What is Dementia?

Dementia is the loss of cognitive functioning; which involves thinking, remembering, and reasoning, and behavioral abilities to the extent that it interferes with a person's daily life and activities. These functions include memory, language skills, visual perception, problem-solving skills, self-management, and the ability to focus and pay attention to things, whether serious or trivial. Some of the things to notice about people with dementia is, they cannot control their emotions, and their personalities may change. Dementia ranges in severity from the mildest stage, when it is just beginning to affect a person's functioning, to the most severe stage, when the person must depend entirely on others for necessary activities of living.

While dementia is more common as people grow older (up to half of all people age 85 or older may have some form of dementia), it is not a normal part of the aging process. This is because many people live into their 90s and beyond without any signs of dementia. One type of dementia, frontotemporal disorders, is more common in middle-aged than older adults. Dementia can also be referred to as major neurocognitive disorder, and it's not a disease itself. Instead, it's a group of symptoms caused by other conditions.

The most common cause of dementia is Alzheimer's disease, and between 60 to 80 percent of people with dementia have Alzheimer's. But there are as many as 50 other causes of dementia. The symptoms that come with dementia may improve with treatment. But many of the diseases that cause dementia are not curable.

Types of Dementia

The common types of dementia include the following:
- **Alzheimer's Disease:** This disease is characterized by what we call plaques, which are found between the dying cells in the brain, and tangles found within the cells of the brain. The presence of the plaques and tangles are to show a form of protein abnormalities in the brain cells structure. The brain tissue of someone living with Alzheimer's disease has fewer nerve cells and connections increasingly, with the total brain size continually shrinking.
- **Mixed Dementia:** This form of dementia shows diagnosis of two or three types occurring together. An example is when a person shows a symptom of Alzheimer's disease and vascular dementia at the same time.
- **Dementia with Lewy Bodies:** It is a neurodegenerative condition that is linked to the abnormalities in the structure of the brain. The brain changes in this situation have involvement of a protein called alpha-synuclein.
- **Parkinson's Disease:** It is a form of dementia that is also marked by the existence of Lewy bodies. In as much as Parkinson's disease is usually considered as a disorder of movement, the symptoms associated with Parkinson can lead to Dementia symptoms.
- **Huntington's Disease:** This form of dementia is characterized by specific types of uncontrolled movements, which also includes dementia.

Other disorders could lead to Dementia symptoms, which includes:

- **Normal Pressure Hydrocephalus:** This occurs when excess cerebrospinal fluid accumulates in the brain.

- **Frontotemporal Dementia:** This type of dementia is also known as Pick's disease.

- **Posterior Cortical Atrophy:** This resembles changes noticed in Alzheimer's disease, but it occurs in a different part of the brain.

- **Down Syndrome:** This is a disease that affects the younger folks, and it increases the likelihood of young-onset Alzheimer's.

Alzheimer's is the most common type of dementia, which is known to make up of up to 50% – 80% of the cases of dementia. Like Alzheimer's disease, Dementia disease is also a disease that could be exhibited as a resultant effect of aging. This is because it makes seniors highly susceptible to the condition called dementia. It is possible to have the existence of more than one type of dementia in the same person. From a global view, dementia has affected an estimated population of 47.5 million people worldwide. From this population, about 10% of the people develop the disease at some point in their lives, although it becomes more prevalent with age. About 3% of the people have dementia between the ages of 65 – 74 years, 19% have dementia between the ages of 75 -84 years, while close to 50% of those over the age of 85 years have dementia. According to Alzheimer's society, there are around a population of 850,000 people living with Dementia in the United Kingdom, and it is projected that by 2025, the number of people living with dementia in the UK will have increased to around 1 million. An analysis conducted from the most recent census in the United States shows that 4.7 million people were living with Alzheimer's disease (a prominent type of dementia). It should also be noted that there one new case of dementia is diagnosed every 4 seconds; and in as much dementia is not a normal part of aging, the sets of people that it affects most are the older people.

Causes of Dementia

If you would agree with me, to any effect of an action, there are always causes resulting in that action. This is the same way some noted causes could be responsible for dementia, and mind you, dementia can be caused by the death of brain cell, and neurodegenerative disease. We cannot say for now if dementia causes the death of brain cells, or death of brain cell causes dementia. Dementia can be caused by the following:

- **Vascular Dementia:** This is also called multi-infarct Dementia. It happens as a result of the death of brain cells caused by such a condition as a cerebrovascular disease; an example of this is a stroke. It prevents normal blood flow, depriving brain cells of oxygen.

- **Injury:** Injury is a causal agent of post-traumatic dementia that is directly linked to the death of brain cell. Some types of traumatic brain injury – most especially repetitive ones such the ones acquired from sporting activities by sportsmen have been related to some forms of dementia happening to them later in life.

Other causes of dementia include:

- **Prion Diseases:** Example of this is Creutzfekdt-Jakob disease. https://www.cdc.gov/prions/index.html
- **HIV Infection:** There is no certainty to how the virus damages the brain, but it is identified to ensue.

Stages and Associated Symptoms of Dementia

The stages and associated symptoms of dementia are grouped into four stages, which includes:

- **Mild Cognitive Impairment:** This stage is characterized by general forgetfulness. This stage affects many people as they age, this, however, progresses to dementia for some people.

- **Mild Dementia:** It is observed that people living with dementia at this stage will experience cognitive impairments that occasionally affects their daily life. Symptoms in this stage include confusion, memory loss, getting lost, personality changes, and difficulty in planning and carrying out tasks.

- **Moderate Dementia:** At this stage, daily life for people living with dementia becomes more challenging, and Dementia patients at this phase need more help than ever before. Symptoms at this stage are similar to mild dementia, only that those symptoms become intense. You might need to help the senior in your care get dressed and even comb their hair. Changes in personality may also occur at this stage; they will start getting suspicious and unnecessarily agitated for no reason. Sleep disturbances also happen at this stage.

- **Severe Dementia:** This is the final stage of dementia, and at this stage, symptoms get considerably worsened. There may be an impairment in communication, and at this point, the patient needs full-time care. Bladder control may be lost and sitting and holding one's head up becomes difficult. What happens in the long run for anyone at this stage of dementia is death. It is only a matter of time.

The general symptoms associated with dementia include the following:

- **Difficulty completing accustomed tasks:** People living dementia often find it arduous to do regular duties that they used to, examples involve cooking a meal, making a drink, or cleaning the house.
- **Recent memory loss:** This symptom might be accompanied by the patient asking the same question that had already been answered repeatedly. This is because the retentive memory that used to be there before now is lost.
- **Misplacing things:** People living with dementia at this stage often forget where they place everyday items such as phones, keys, or wallets.
- **Problems with abstract thinking:** They are always not putting their thoughts in place, people these symptoms often have issues when it comes to dealing with money.
- **Communication problems:** This symptom goes in line with the Dementia patients having a speech impairment, forgetting simple words, wrong use of words, and difficulty with language.
- **Loss of initiative:** They don't show interest in getting things done; they are always laid back and not wanting to initiate a course of action that could involve starting something or going somewhere.
- **Personality changes:** This symptom shows people used to know to start exhibiting some attitudes that would make you doubt whether you still recognize them or not. They become irritable, suspicious, fearful, and they lack empathy.
- **Mood swings:** They often switch moods unexpectedly and surprisingly. You notice an unexplained change in their outlook or temper.

Diagnosis of Dementia

It is like Alzheimer's; there is no one test to determine whether someone has dementia. Medical doctors diagnose dementia based on a careful examination of the medical history, physical examination, laboratory tests, specific changes in thinking, daily function, and behavior associated with each Dementia type. Dementia is examined by medical doctors based on a high level of certainty. However, it is more tasking to determine the dementia. This is as a result of the fact that the symptoms and brain changes associated with dementia can overlap. For some situations, a doctor may diagnose the disease dementia without mentioning the dementia that the diagnosis belongs.

It has been shown from studies that dementia cannot be reliably diagnosed without using the standard tests below. After fully completing them, and recording all the answers, then the diagnosis can be made effectively. The cognitive Dementia tests include some standard intentional questions which are asked below:

- What is your age?
- What is the year?
- What is the time, to the nearest hour?
- What is the name of the hospital where you are present?
- What is your date of birth?
- Can you recognize these people, for example, a family, the doctor, the nurse, or a caregiver?
- Who is the president of your country?
- What is your address?
- Repeat an address of the test that I will give you now (for example, 21, Kensington drive).
- Count in descending order from 20 down to 1.

The results from gathered from these questions are going to be a significant determinant of giving a correct diagnosis of the presence and the stage of the disease.

Effects of Dementia

The effects of dementia are on the seniors is the same as that of Alzheimer's, wouldn't be wrong to revise it again under this section, would it? Now let's see how bad it could be on the seniors.

1. **Speaking, reading, and writing impairment:** They start to have issues with speaking; it affects their speech pattern; they now find it difficult to speak well. Reading books that used to be an easy thing or hobby gradually becomes a difficulty. Also, writing becomes an issue for seniors as a result of dementia.

2. **Their Personality and Behavioral pattern are affected:** This disease turns our seniors to become who they were not in the earlier phases of their lives. A wholly friendly and confident person over time changes to become a person with irregular mood changes; obsessive, compulsive, or socially unacceptable behavior; loss of interest, motivation, or initiative; loss of empathy among others. You must understand that this is not who they are; instead, this is what dementia have turned them to become.

3. **Reasoning Impairment:** This comes with difficulty to think of common words while speaking, including a hesitant speech; the sense of judgment becomes affected, and errors are made with speech, spellings, and writings.

4. **Impaired visuospatial abilities:** This comes with their inability to identify faces of people and everyday objects, it also comes with failure to make use of simple tools, an

example of this is putting on your clothes in the wrong way.

5. **Retentive Impairment:** Dementia disease comes with a drastically reduced ability to take in new information, with difficulty in remembering previous events. What will you say about a person who couldn't recall the sweet memories of his/her wedding day? What about the circumstances surrounding the birth of her first child? Seniors living with dementia start to misplace personal belongings, forget appointments and events, get lost on a familiar route, and repeat conversations and questions uncontrollably.

6. **Getting shunned by loved ones:** This here is common with people living around seniors that have dementia. They try as much as possible to avoid them and even take them away from the society of people. Doing this usually, make things worse for the senior. Neglecting them is not always the best at this stage of their lives.

7. **Death:** This is the end of it all, sooner or later, deterioration will set, and the resultant effect is always death.

The Control of Dementia

It is crucial for us to know that the death of brain cells is irreversible, and as of now, there has been no stated cure for the degenerative disease. Now what we need to know here is how to manage the situation so that it will not make things difficult for our seniors, thereby making life unbearable for them. The disease can be controlled if we are ready and committed to going through the control measures.

We need to watch our seniors closely at this point to make sure they are not indulging in habits that can worsen their condition. Habits like smoking, alcohol should be put under severe check. They need proper care at this point and undivided attention. Medical therapies can also be used to mild the effects of the disease on our seniors, always consult with your physician to ensure correct prescriptions.

Brain training is another mechanism that may help to improve the cognitive functioning, and help deal with a forgetfulness which is likened to the early stages. Devices like mnemonics and other memory aids such as computer recall devices might also be of help.

Different therapeutic interventions are always employed to make things easier for our seniors living with dementia. Some of them include getting them enrolled in activities and daycare programs, involvement in support groups where they will meet other patients like themselves. This would go a long way in making them feel loved and make them realize that they are not alone on this journey.

Chapter Five
Transforming Mental Illness To Mental Wellness

Transforming mental illness into mental wellness, what comes to mind? Do you see it as just a mere exercise, or you see as some laid down steps to take, or you see as a way of life to imbibe? All of these could be true. However, we need to have a complete understanding of what it takes for something to transform for the better, or the other way around.

Defining transformation could come in the form of seeing it as a gradual or drastic change that happens to a person or something over some time. When transformation takes place in something or someone, it is to make us know that there is a shift from a phase of 'what used to be' to 'what is' Also, there could be a transformation from what is back to the initial stage of what used to be.

Now looking at it from the human context, and taking into consideration the topical issue at hand, any human that used to be in good health but along the line, a shift took place, and mental illness crept in; the situation that is noticed there and then is a transformation from a state of mental wellness to mental illness. This is the period when you have someone that used to be okay, friendly, healthy, and in good state of mind becoming some else entirely. They start to act funny, exercise irrational behaviors and exhibit some characters that do not depict someone in a good state of mental health. The things that they show are the symptoms that originate with the type of mental illness that is diagnosed in them, which could be either schizophrenia, bipolar disorder, or dementia, or any other mental illness that is not discussed in the outline of this book. I should bring this to your attention that most of these mental illnesses exhibit one, two, or more similarities in the symptoms that they present. Also, there could be a couple of risk factors that are common to these mental illnesses — distinguishing between which is which among the illnesses are best done by medical experts.

We have looked at the transformation from mental wellness to mental illness, what about looking at it the other way around from mental illness to mental wellness? Let me do a quick definition of mental wellness here – simply put, mental wellness defines a normal and healthy human living condition which comes with a good state of mind, sound cognitive state, proper reasoning, proper coordination, rational decision making, healthy relationship, and appropriate response to the outer environment (physical and human environment). Like I discussed earlier, an impairment in mental health is what transforms one from mental illness to mental wellness. However, it is possible for a restoration process to take place – the restoration process causes a transformation from mental illness back to a state of mental wellness. You want to know how? All you need to do is go through the points outlined below.

Acceptance

One of the mistakes that are often made by people living with one form of mental illness or the other is that they do not want to realize that they have mental illness in the first place. They want to make themselves feel like 'I'm fine,' 'I've got no problems' – when in the real sense there is a process of impairment going on in their metal functioning system. Some of them even argue with their loved ones who have noticed some strange symptoms that they exhibit at one point or the other. Some even decline the offer to take them for a medical checkup. When you do this to yourself, you are doing yourself more harm than good. This is because of the time that you are wasting in arguing and not going for a checkup to get proper treatment, and the symptoms are busy getting advanced in your mental system. You need to be sensitive with your body and act fast whenever you notice something in your body or that of your loved ones before things get out hand.

When you are diagnosed with bipolar disorder, or schizophrenia, or dementia, or any form of mental illness; what you need to do now is not to write yourself off and quit, you need to call yourself to order and come to terms with your present condition. Coming to terms with your current situation deals with getting more knowledge about your diagnosis. You can do this by reading books like the one you are reading right now, going on the internet, or asking questions from the medical experts on the nature of the illness and symptoms that are presented. Getting knowledge about your condition brings to a complete understanding of it, and with that, you can tackle it the best way possible.

Accepting your current condition involves letting the people around you know about your health so that they will not get offended when they notice that you are exhibiting some symptoms occasionally. When they know about what you are going through, they will understand you better and know how to help deal with it.

The process of acceptance involves two sets of people coming to terms with what you are going through. The first person is YOU, you own your body, and your attitude to taking care of your body goes a long way to your healing process. The second person or set of people are your families loved ones; they need to understand that you are going through another phase in your life, they need to realize that the condition that you are facing will require them giving you constant care and support. When you and your loved ones could come to terms to the mental illness you are living, speedy recovery will be assured.

Communication and Interaction

Communication and interaction speed up the process of healing. Communication and interaction take a two-way dimension. The first is you being able to talk to people around about your condition and discussing with your family and loved ones about your needs, and how they could help. This phase of your life is not the time for you to allow your ego to set in and make yourself feel you are self-sufficient. We all need somebody to lean on one point or the other in our lives. Don't make yourself feel like you are a liability to them, because the fact that you need people's help and care doesn't make you a burden. Don't stay alone, staying alone is going to mess with your mind, and it could make matters worse; so, staying in the company of people who love and care for you genuinely is going to go a long way.

The other part to this is targeting the loved ones taking time to communicate to their loved ones living with one mental illness or the other. Proper communication and interaction is a significant way of showing love care and support; you need to know that interacting with them is a form of therapy on its own. When you delight in being around them, what you are making them feel is love, and that could be a motivational force that would speed up their restoration back to a sound state of mental wellness. Proper communication will not make them feel isolated in any way. You need to keep the communication and interaction with loved ones living with one form of mental illness or the other optimized and consistent.

Zoe, 35, a beautiful, intelligent young woman who had her career in the fashion world going well, and people always flocking around her as she was a sought out too many. Years into her career, she started noticing some weird changes in herself, coupled with the fact that her sister; Trish, 30, had been complaining about her recent changes in her manner of behavior which she never believed. This caused a strained relationship between herself and her sister, who was all she got. Things started going down with her, and her career began to dwindle. It was at that point that she discovered she was going to go for a medical checkup. On getting to the hospital for a medical appointment, she was diagnosed with bipolar disorder. This was terrible news for her, and she felt so stigmatized. She started avoiding people because she didn't want them to know that she has a mental illness. She started indulging in alcohol and drugs. Time went by, and things went from bad to worse, she fell into depression, and she committed suicide when she felt she couldn't bear it anymore. The news got to Trish as a shocking one; they have not been communicating in a while. Although Trish couldn't forgive herself for staying away from her sister thinking, she developed new bad habits. She could have been patient enough to communicate with her. But the deed is done, and the lesson was learned in a hard way. Let us be patient enough to communicate and interact with our loved ones living with a mental illness, and patients should always speak out. We can help each other to become better when we are vocal about our struggles.

Management and Care

It is essential for you to know that after taking your time to study your loved ones and getting your facts about their health condition, the next step for you is to put a well-structured management pattern in place, which will make things easy for you while adapting to the state of their health. Managing the situation involves informing the people around you of the condition that you or your loved one is facing for them to understand the position of things around them. And, for them to know how to interact with those affected with the mental illness; informing people around you about their health condition will make them not take offenses at any character they exhibit as a result of their illness. It also involves structuring a caregiving schedule that will be effective and less stressful for you. For instance, let's say you have a time demanding job and your affected loved one living with you, and, I know you wouldn't want to lose the job that puts food on the table as a result of taking yourself or loved one. In this situation, you can employ the services of a trained caregiver that is competent enough to take good care of them. However, that is not a good excuse for you not to spend quality time with them. Make sure you plan your time well, so you could have your time giving care apart from the ones your caregiver would provide. When you do this, you are going to bring them to a phase of a speedy recovery.

Let me tell you a brief story of **Papa San, 82**, who is loved by everyone in his community due to his active nature when it comes to getting things done. He was a goal getter, always making sure he does everything it takes within his capacity to get tasks done excellently. He never quits. His sense of humor was second to none; this makes his grandchildren and the kids living around him always enjoy every moment they spend with him. His knowledge of sound judgment makes him preferable compared to a host of other people of his age group living in the community; whenever you come for advice from Papa San, be sure you are going to leave his place with a sound mind to make the right decisions, that's how he is or should I say how good he was? He was never alone; always in the company of different people; either those he mentors or with the kids coming around to have a good time with him. He was such a lovely soul. It happened that her daughter, **Tasha, 55**, started noticing some changes in her father, which is quite unusual with the Papa San that she use to know. She noticed him suddenly started forgetting pieces of stuff, he could keep cellphone on the cabinet in the kitchen, and the next minute he is already looking for it all over the living room arguing that he left it on the table. Tasha was putting these things to mind, but she didn't consider them as something dangerous. Things took a drastic turn when her father got missing on her way to the Grocery store, and he was later found in another neighborhood by the police after she had filed a report to the police department. All Papa could say when he was found was, he missed his way. Tasha was surprised at the sudden change.

"Common Dad, you've always been going to this grocery store since I was 10," Tasha said, worried sick that something terrible had happened to her father. It dawned on her at this point that she needed to take Papa San to the hospital for urgent medical attention. After running some critical examinations by the doctor, he was diagnosed with Middle-stage Alzheimer's – a profound type of dementia. That was terrible news for Tasha, who is a practicing nurse. Due to her profession, she was able to give proper care to her father, she made her kids and the people around her in the community to understand Papa San's condition and the character that he could be exhibiting under these conditions. The people understood him and were able to give him all the love and support you could ever imagine. Papa San was always in the company of people, although at times he withdraws himself from those visiting to be on his own, still the support and attention he got from his loved ones never decreased. Papa San was able to live for a couple more years before he finally passed away at the age of 87.

We could notice from this story that the sensitivity of his daughter made her able to see a change in her father, and was able to understand what to do, and how to handle the situation when she was diagnosed. She knew at that point that it is of utmost importance to study him to understand the ways and manner of handling the peculiarity that comes with his condition. Like it is the work of a psychologist to study human behavior, you need to be sensitive and be calm enough at this point to take time and examine your loved ones living with any form of mental illness. It was easy for Tasha to adapt because she took her time to study the peculiarity of her father's mental illness and the symptoms that he exhibits, and she was able to understand and manage her father's condition well. So, please take your time to study your loved ones so that you can easily adapt to their health conditions, for them to get the love they deserve from you. Also, the patients should try and cooperate with their loved ones.

Recovery

The next step after proper communication and management is put in place is recovery. The recovery process is more like a journey that could be easy when there is cooperation between the person affected and the caregivers. The affected patients need to go to the hospital from time to time for proper check-ups. And for those having a mental illness that is not curable, they need to manage it well by using the prescribed drugs in a proportionate pattern.

Attending support group meetings will also enable them to see people with similar issues and discussing how they got through with it; this will make them feel they are not alone. Getting help from relevant agencies for job provision will push depression away. When all the therapies are put in place, be sure of an optimized recovery.

Summary

From everything discussed in the beginning, it is crucial to understand that mental illness is real, and it happens to people around us. The technique and manner we approach it goes a long way towards achieving restored mental health or a well-managed condition. There is more expected from those living with the ailment, and there are expectations from the caregivers in their approach to handling the symptoms exhibited. Sensitivity and patience are vital, and mental wellness is always the goal.

The Journey is Eternal!!

www.ingramcontent.com/pod-product-compliance
Lightning Source LLC
Chambersburg PA
CBHW021907170526
45157CB00005B/2009